Mental Health/Substance Abuse Assessment Guide

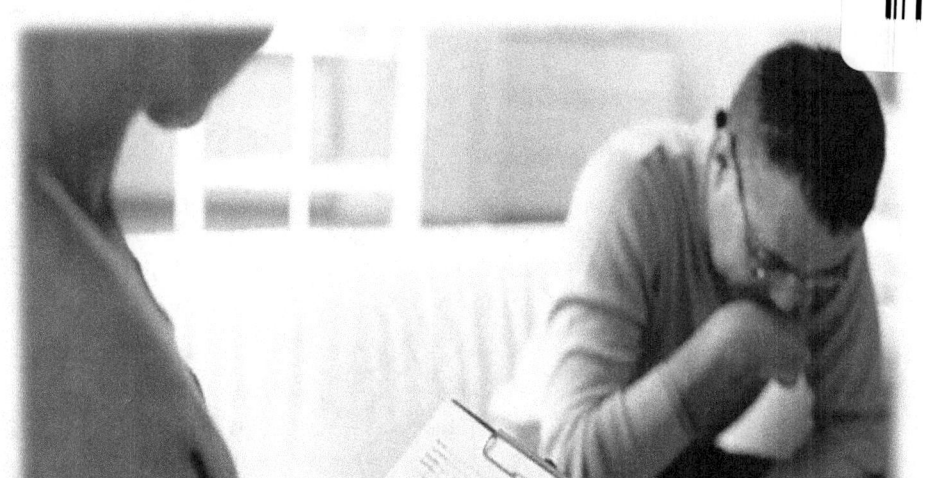

A Comprehensive, Multi-Modal Approach
to Screening and Identifying Client Needs

Developed by Ramsey Bradley, M.S.

Cautionary Note and Disclaimer

Please note that when you use any of the words, phrases, descriptors, sentences, and/or procedures described in the Mental Health/Substance Abuse Assessment Guide, you are assuming full responsibility for all consequences-clinical, legal, ethical and financial. The author(s) cannot, do not, and will not assume any responsibility for their use or implication in your practice or with any patient or client. Additionally, the author(s) shall not be liable in the event of incidental or consequential damages in regards to or rising out of any use by the user of the materials outlined in the Guide.

By employing the Mental Health/Substance Abuse Assessment Guide the user also signifies his/her acceptance of the limits of the work and his/her acceptance of completed personal responsibility for all such uses.

Furthermore, the author(s) presume (1) that the user of the Mental Health/Substance Abuse Assessment Guide is qualified by education and/or training to employ it ethically and legally and (2) that the user of the Assessment Guide not exceed the limits of documentable competence in his/her discipline as indicated by the codes of ethical practice.

Introduction

Identification of most psychological disorders require an all inclusive Multi-modal Treatment Assessment. Since many clients also suffer from dual substance abuse, mental health, occupational, health, and/or social problems make their disorders much more difficult to treat. This Multi-modal coordinated effort provides for a comprehensive range of services including counseling, case management, medications, housing, vocational rehabilitation, social skills training, as well as, family interventions that are modified to include both diagnosis.

The Mental Health/Substance Abuse Assessment Guide will help in the following areas:

- It serves as a guide to help organize your thoughts when writing, to ensure that you have addressed all of the relevant topics.
- It can structure a report to make certain that you haven't missed anything of importance.
- It can suggest individual goals, objectives and therapeutic interventions to help personalize a report or description.
- Also, the planner is organized in a manner that you can actually do a mini-mental status examination by selecting from the offered questions.

The use of this Mental Health/Substance Abuse Assessment Guide will assist the clinically competent professional in carrying out his/her report writing tasks and at the same time making sure that they are writing better, more comprehensive reports.

In closing, I would like to personally thank you for your interest and consideration in choosing the Mental Health/Substance Abuse Assessment Guide.

Ramsey Bradley, M.S.
Program Developer

Contents

- Anger
- Antisocial Personality Disorder
- Anxiety- General
- Attention Deficit/Hyper. Disorder, NOS
- Borderline Personality Disorder
- Dependent Personality Disorder
- Depression, NOS
- Dissociative Disorder, NOS
- Eating Disorder, NOS
- Expressive Language Disorder
- Impulsivity
- Legal Issues
- Language Disorder
- Living Arrangement
- Mathematics Disorder
- Medical Issues
- Memory Challenges, NOS
- Obsessive Compulsive Disorder
- Occupational Problems

The Intake Process

The therapist, intake worker, or receptionist who has first contact with a prospective client should do everything possible to facilitate entry into treatment. Staff should provide timely assistance and be flexible in scheduling, empathic when appropriate, and optimistic about the client's ability to change. This will help the therapist or intake worker provide the friendly, respectful, and flexible treatment access required. All initial contacts can be handled by a receptionist or clinician.

Once the client contacts the clinic to request treatment (either by telephone or by walking in), every effort should be made to conduct the intake interview as soon as possible. At least three studies show that scheduling intake appointments with minimal delay significantly reduces the attrition rate between initial contact and the intake appointment.

Ideally, the intake would be done the same day; if that is not possible, then try to schedule it within 24 hours. The least accommodating schedule should be within 2 working days of contact, although occasionally this process may take longer.

Be prepared to be flexible on timing and scheduling. If the client cannot stay for the complete intake, schedule another appointment as soon as possible to complete the process. However, a brief introductory meeting with a therapist is recommended at the end of the initial intake session even if the intake needs to be completed in a second session.

If clients bring a spouse or partner to intake, it is important to make the partner feel comfortable if they are going to participate with treatment.

However, the assessment interview is conducted with the client only. Prior to and after the assessment, inform the partner about the assessment and treatment process. If appropriate, raise the possibility of relationship counseling and encourage it at this time. The intake session is one of the most important elements of the treatment process. This may be the first treatment experience for many client's, and they may feel somewhat uncomfortable or ambivalent about being there. Some client's may have had an unpleasant treatment experience in the past and are somewhat wary of treatment in general.

It is important that clients are made to feel as comfortable as possible during the intake process.

• Be aware of the client's potential uneasiness and do everything possible to make the initial meeting a positive experience.
• Convey positive, can-do messages. The client should clearly hear that, by working together, the client and clinic staff can resolve problems that brought the individual to treatment.
• Accommodate the need for brief breaks, food or drink, or need to make a phone call.

It is also important to collect detailed information on the severity of the client's presenting issues, treatment readiness, current psychiatric functioning, medical problems, employment, legal issues, and family and social problems.

The Evaluation Process

- Engage and support the client

- Complete appropriate client authorizations, identify and contact collaterals such as family, friends, and other treatment providers to gather additional information.

- Screen for and detect dual-diagnosis

- Determine severity of dual-diagnosis

- Determine appropriate care setting (inpatient/outpatient)

- Determine functional impairment

- Identify strengths and supports

- Identify cultural, spiritual and support needs

- Identify additional areas of concern (health, housing, vocational, educational, cognitive, social, or spiritual, etc).

- Determine level of readiness for change

- Prepare intervention plan

The Mental Status Examination (MSE)

A Mental State Examination (MSE) is an assessment of a patient's current level of cognitive (knowledge-related) ability, appearance, emotional mood, and speech and thought patterns at the time of evaluation. The purpose of a mental status examination is to assess the presence and extent of a person's mental impairment at the time of screening.

At first all this might seem overwhelming and time consuming, but really it's not that bad to do. It can generally be done in a few minutes when you need to do specific things, and the vast majority of this you can get from interviewing and simply watching the client carefully.

The Functional Behavioral Assessment

The Functional Behavioral Assessment is based on the idea that the therapist must address multiple modalities of an individual to identify and treat all mental and/or substance abuse disorders. According The Functional Behavioral Assessment, all individuals are affected in different ways and in different amounts by each dimension of personality, and should be treated accordingly for treatment to be successful. The Assessment sees individuals as products of interaction between genetic endowment, physical environment, and social learning history.

The Functional Behavioral Assessment starts after the client has been assessed based on his/her emotional responses, sensory displays and the manner in which he/she interacts with people around through behavior, effect, sensations, images, cognition, drugs and interpersonal activities.

Based on this assessment, the therapist will introduce the client to the first screening session. During this time, the therapist and the client will create a list of problems and the appropriate treatments that may suit him/her the most. Since the treatment is based upon individual cases, each remedial strategy is considered as an effective method for the clients.

Post the completion of the initial assessment, a more detailed diagnosis is done using questionnaires and checklist. The therapist shall diagnose both the actual profile as well as the structural profile of the client. Such a diagnosis will define the target which both the therapist and the client would want to achieve once the treatment is complete.

The Functional Behavioral Assessment is a flexible manner of therapy since each treatment plan is devised keeping all possibilities in mind.

16

The Mental Status Exam (MSE)

Patient Name: _____ Date of MSE: _____

Appearance: Attitude		Normal	Cooperative
		Abnormal	Uncooperative, Hostile, Guarded, Suspicious
Mood		Euthymic	calm, comfortable, euthymic, friendly, pleasant, unremarkable
		Angry	angry, belligerent, confrontational, frustrated, hostile, impatient, irritable, oppositional, outraged
		Euphoric	cheerful, ecstatic, elated, euphoric, giddy, happy, jovial
		Dysphoric	despondent, distraught, dysphoric, grieving, hopeless, lugubrious, overwhelmed, remorseful, sad
		Apprehensive	anxious, apprehensive, fearful, frightened, high-stung, nervous, overwhelmed, panicked, tense, terrified, worried
Affect	Appropriateness	normal	appropriate, congruent
		abnormal	inappropriate incongruent
	Intensity	normal	normal
		abnormal	blunted, exaggerated, flat, heightened, overly dramatic
	Variability/ Mobility	normal	mobile
		abnormal	constricted, fixed, immobile, labile
	Range	normal	full
		abnormal	restricted range
	Reactivity	normal	reactive, responsive
		abnormal	nonreactive, nonresponsive

Speech		Fluency, repetition, comprehension, naming, writing, reading, prosody, quality of speech.	Comment specifically
Thought	Process	Disorders of Connectedness	circumstantiality, flight of ideas, loose associations, tangentiality, word salad, thought blocking
	Content	thoughts	delusions, homicidal ideation, magical thinking, obsessions, overvalued ideas, paranoia, phobia, poverty of speech, preoccupations, ruminations, suicidal ideation, suspiciousness
		perceptions	autoscopy, déjà vu, depersonalization, derealization, hallucinations, illusion

Functional Behavioral Assessment: Part 1 (Description)

Student Name: _____ ID: _____ DOB: _____

Data Sources (Please check all that apply):

☐ Observation | ☐ Student Interview | ☐ Teacher Interview |

☐ Parent Interview | ☐ Rating Scales | ☐ Normative Testing

Description of Behavior (No. _____):
Setting(s) in which behavior occurs:
Frequency:
Intensity (Consequences of problem behavior on student, peers, instructional environment):
Duration:
Describe Previous Interventions:
Educational impact:

Functional Behavioral Assessment: Part 2 (Function)

Name: _____   Date: _____

Function of Behavior (No. _____): Specify hypothesized function for each area checked below.
☐ *Affective Regulation/Emotional Reactivity* (Identify emotional factors; anxiety, depression, anger, poor self-concept; that play a role in organizing or directing problem behavior):
☐ *Cognitive Distortion* (Identify distorted thoughts; inaccurate attributions, negative self-statements, erroneous interpretations of events; that play a role in organizing or directing problem behavior):

☐ *Reinforcement* (Identify environmental triggers and payoffs that play a role in organizing and directing problem behavior):
  Antecedents:
  Consequences:

☐ *Modeling* (Identify the degree to which the behavior is copied, who they are copying the behavior from, and why they are copying the behavior):
☐ *Family Issues* (Identify family issues that play a part in organizing and directing problem behavior):
☐ *Physiological/Constitutional* (Identify physiological and/or personality characteristics; developmental disabilities, temperament; that play a part in organizing and directing problem behavior):
☐ *Communicate need* (Identify what the student is trying to say through the problem behavior):
☐ *Curriculum/Instruction* (Identify how instruction, curriculum, or educational environment play a part in organizing and directing problem behavior):

Client Intake Form

CLIENT INFORMATION

Name: _____   Date: _____

Client Identification Number: _____ Social Security Number: _____ - ____ - _____

Mailing Address: _____City: _____State: _____Zip: _____

Telephone Number: (_____) _____-_____   Email: _____

Date of Birth: ___/___/_____ Age: _____ Sex: _____Race: _____ Religion: _____

Ethnicity: _____   Citizenship: _____

Emergency Contact Name: _____

_____

Relationship: _____

_____

Mailing Address: _____City: _____State: _____Zip: _____

Telephone Number: (_____) _____-_____   Email: _____

Comments:_____

REFERRAL SOURCE INFORMATION

Referral Source: _____

_____

Referral Contact Name: _____

_____

Telephone Number: (___) ____-_____Fax Number: (___)____-_____Email: _____

Mailing Address: _____City: _____State: _____Zip: ____

Client Identification Number for referral _____

Comments: _____

_____

HEALTH INSURANCE INFORMATION

Health Insurance Company Name:
_____

Type: _____

Name(s) Insured: _____ Contact Number: _____

Policy Number: _____ Contact Number: _____

Group Number: _____ Telephone Number: _____

Other Information:
_____

Comments:_____

SOCIAL WELFARE INFORMATION

SSDI Number:
_____

Medicare Number/Medicaid Number:
_____

RELATIONSHIP AND FAMILY HISTORY INFORMATION

Were you raised by both parents? ____yes ____no, if no please explain:
_____

What was "growing up" like for you as a child?
_____

Did any member of your childhood family use or abuse alcohol and or drugs? _____yes _____no, if yes please explain:

What were the primary ethnic, cultural beliefs of your childhood family? Please explain:
_____

What was the social and economic status of your childhood family? Please explain: _____

CURRENT FAMILY:

How would you describe your current living conditions?

_____

Describe your current sexual orientation: _____ Describe your current sex life: _____

Has any member of your current family been negatively affected by your alcohol and or drug abuse?
_____yes _____no,

if yes, please explain who has been most effected and in what way: _____

Do you believe that your family members will support you in your recovery? _____yes _____no, if
yes, please explain who might be most supportive and the type of support: _____

Do you have any specific cultural beliefs or practices that might effect this assessment process,
treatment or your recovery?: _____yes _____no, if yes, please explain: _____

How would you describe your current religious or spiritual beliefs? _____

EDUCATIONAL:

What is your highest grade level completed?: _____

Do you have any difficulty with reading, writing or comprehension?: _____yes _____no, if yes, please
explain:_____

Do you speak and or comprehend a language other than English?: _____yes _____no, if yes, please
explain:

_____

Have you ever experienced problems in school because of your alcohol and or drug abuse problem?:
_____yes _____no, if yes, please explain: _____

VOCATIONAL.

Do you have any special employment skills? ____yes ____no, if yes, please explain: _____

Are you currently employed?:_____yes _____no, if yes, please explain: _____

Have you ever had an accident or injury on the job because of your alcohol and or drug abuse
problem? ____ yes ____no, if yes, please explain: _____

Have you ever been fired or laid off from a job because of your alcohol and or drug abuse problem?:
_____yes _____no, if yes, please explain: _____

RECREATIONAL/ LEISURE

Describe your recreational and leisure interests and activities: _____

When was the last time you engaged in recreational or leisure activities?:_____

What effect has your alcohol and or drug abuse had on your recreational or leisure activities?:
_____

LEGAL INFORMATION

Have you ever been arrested for a civil or criminal offense; including an alcohol or drug related offense?:__yes __no. If yes, please explain date by years, type of charges, and outcome:_____

Are you currently or have you ever been ordered by the civil or criminal courts to alcohol / drug abuse / mental health treatment?: _____yes _____no, if yes, please explain date by years, type of treatment, and outcome:_____

Are you currently or have you ever been on probation?: _____yes _____no, if yes, please explain date by years, name, address, telephone number of officer: _____

Are you currently awaiting charges, court hearing or sentencing?: _____yes _____no, if yes, please explain charges, court dates: _____

MEDICAL INFORMATION

How would you rate your current physical health: ____poor ___good ____very good ___excellent ___

Comments:_____

Do you have any chronic medical problems? _____ yes _____ no, if yes please explain:
_____

Do you currently take any prescribed medications? _____yes _____ no, if yes, please list the name(s)of the medication, how much and how often taken:
_____

Do you have a primary care physician? _____ yes _____ no, if yes please list the doctors name, address, telephone number: _____

Do you believe that your alcohol and or drug abuse problem(s) have had a negative impact on your physical health? _____yes _____no, if yes please explain: _____

Do you have any medical or dental problems that require immediate special attention or could prevent your participation in treatment? ____yes ___no, if yes please explain: _____

ALCOHOL / DRUG ABUSE INFORMATION

Do you believe that you have a problem with alcohol and or drug abuse problem?: _____yes _____no, If yes, please explain: _____

Please identify if you have ever used or abused alcohol and or the drugs listed as follows:

Alcohol: ____ _____ Age Started _____Age Ended _____ Route _____Quantity

Comments:

_____

Narcotics: _____ _____ Age Started _____Age Ended _____ Route _____Quantity

Comments:

_____

Barbiturates: ____ _____ Age Started _____Age Ended _____ Route _____Quantity

Comments:

_____

Tranquilizers: ____ _____ Age Started _____Age Ended _____ Route _____Quantity

Comments:

_____

Cocaine: _____ _____ Age Started _____Age Ended _____ Route _____Quantity

Comments:

_____

Amphetamines: ____ _____ Age Started _____Age Ended _____ Route _____Quantity

Comments:

_____

Marijuana: _____ _____ Age Started _____Age Ended _____ Route _____Quantity

Comments:

_____

Hallucinogens: _____ _____ Age Started _____ Age Ended _____ Route _____ Quantity

Comments:

_____

Inhalants: _____ _____ Age Started _____ Age Ended _____ Route _____ Quantity

Comments:

_____

Nicotine: _____ _____ Age Started _____ Age Ended _____ Route _____ Quantity

Comments:

_____

Other Drugs: _____ _____ Age Started _____ Age Ended _____ Route _____ Quantity

Comments:

_____

Please list your primary alcohol/drug of choice: _____First; _____ Second; _____Third

As a result of your use and or abuse of alcohol and or drugs have you ever experienced any consequences in any area of your major life domains?: ____yes ___no, if yes, please explain:

_____

Physical: _____ Blackouts _____ Withdrawal _____ Tolerance ____ Chronic Illness

Other:_____

Mental: _____ Obsessive Thought _____ Compulsive Behavior _____ Confused Thinking

Other:_____

Emotional: _____ Depression _____ Angry Outbursts ____Guilt ____ Mood Swings

Other:

_____

Social: _____ Relationship Problems _____ Social Isolation ____ Marital Problems

Other: _____

Spiritual: _____ Value Conflicts _____ Immoral Behaviors _____ Stopped Spiritual Practice

Other:_____

Have you ever received treatment for an alcohol and or drug abuse problem?: _____ yes _____ no, if yes please list the dates by years, type of treatment programs, reason for treatment and discharge status: _____

Do you believe that any of your previous treatment has helped you? _____ yes _____ no, if yes please explain: _____

What do you believe are your strengths and weaknesses related to your potential for completion of treatment and recovery? _____

Are you aware of any persons, places or things that may "trigger" your relapse to active use of alcohol and or drugs?: _____ yes _____ no, if yes, please identify the most significant triggers to your relapse:

_____

MENTAL HEALTH INFORMATION

Have you ever received counseling or treatment for emotional, mental health or family issues?: _____ yes _____ no, if yes, explain dates by years, type of treatment for counseling, reason for counseling, discharge status: _____

Have you ever been prescribed psychotropic medications for emotional, mental health or family issues?: _____ yes _____ no, if yes, please explain the dates by years, name of psychiatrist, type of medication, reason for medication, reason for continued or discontinued use: _____

Have you ever had suicidal ideas, thoughts or tried to commit suicide? _____ yes _____ no, if yes, please explain dates by years, plan, circumstances: _____

Has anyone in your childhood or current family ever been treated for emotional or mental health issues?: ____ yes _____ no, if yes, please explain dates by years, what family member, reason for treatment, current or discharge status: _____

Have you ever been physically, sexually or emotionally abused as a child or adult?: ____ yes _____ no, if yes, please explain age, type of abuse, circumstances, consequences: _____

Have you ever physically, sexually or emotionally abused a child or an adult?: _____ yes _____ no, if yes, please explain age, type of abuse, circumstances, consequences: _____

DIAGNOSTIC IMPRESSION: DSM-IV Diagnostic Impression

AXIS 1.

_____

AXIS 2.

_____

AXIS 3.

_____

AXIS 4.

_____

AXIS 5.

_____

ICD-9 DIAGNOSTIC IMPRESSION:
Covered codes if applicable:

Primary ICD-9 Diagnosis __ __ __ . __ __ _____

Secondary ICD-9 Diagnosis __ __ __ . __ __ _____

TREATMENT PLANNING NEEDS:

Medical Goals and Objectives needed in treatment planning? ___ Yes ___ No

Psychiatric Goals and Objectives needed in treatment planning? ___ Yes ___ No

CLINICAL SUMMARY (Clinicians interpretation of the Bio-psychosocial assessment):

_____

_____

_____

_____

_____

_____

_____

TREATMENT RECOMMENDATIONS. (Indicate initial treatment and all subsequent treatment as necessary)

_____

_____

_____

_____

_____

_____

_____

_____

_____

_____

SIGNATURES

Client: _____Date: _____
              (Name)

Counselor: _____Date: _____
            (Name, Title, & Credentials)

Qualified Supervisor: _____Date: _____
              (Name, Title, & Credentials)

Multimodal Therapy

Introduction

Multimodal Therapy is based on the need for customized treatments depending on the client. The therapist can use various treatment modals by asking what is best for the individual. The foundation is social learning and communication theories in which the therapist acknowledges BASIC ID: affective responses, sensory reactions, images, cognitions, interpersonal relationships and drugs.

- **Behavior:** What specific action do you want to do more of/ less of?
- **Affect:** What emotion would you like to increase or decrease?
- **Sensation:** What sensation would you like to have more often or experience less frequently?
- **Imagery:** What mental picture would you like "see" more often or less often in your "mind's eye?"
- **Cognition:** What specific thought would you like to increase or decrease; start or stop?
- **Interpersonal relationships:** What specific social change would you like to make?
- **Drugs/Health/ Biology:** What specific change in a health habit or physical issue would you like to make?

  To illustrate, here is an example:
- **Behavior:** Take more walks after dinner instead of watching TV
- **Affect**: Reduce stress and anxiety
- **Sensation:** Experience less muscle tension
- **Imagery:** Visualize more success
- **Cognition:** Reduce self-criticism and increase self-affirmations
- **Interpersonal:** Spend more time with friends
- **Drugs/Health:** Eat more vegetables and less processed food

These are known as modalities and when they are all addressed the client can be assessed while the therapist builds a customized treatment plan. It is based on recognizing mental conditions and how they affect the personal responses and emotions.

The goal of Multimodal Therapy is to create customized treatment for each client depending on their psychological or behavioral problems. When therapists can recognize that each patient has a different way of thinking and feeling they will be more successful in treating the patient's disorder. At times Multimodal Therapy may also focus on the physiological conditions that the patient is experiencing through combined treatments if necessary. Since the treatment can be catered to each strategy the overall method is effective.

The MMT Treatment Plan below will help you identify helpful changes you and your client can make in order to have a positive impact on their own mental wellbeing.

Multi-modal Treatment Plan

Modality	Problem	Plan
Behavior: Actions, coping strategies, reactions, what I do, what I avoid doing		Do less of, or stop: Do more of, or start:
Affect / Emotions: What I feel emotionally E.g. depressed, angry, anxious, stressed, sad. What makes me feel this way?		Do less of, or stop: Do more of, or start:
Sensation: See, hear, taste, smell, touch, pain, tension, sexuality		Do less of, or stop: Do more of, or start:
Imagery: Thinking in pictures, self image, fantasies		Do less of, or stop: Do more of, or start:
Cognition: Thoughts, attitudes, beliefs, values, opinions, thinking styles		Do less of, or stop: Do more of, or start:
Interpersonal: Communicating and being with others, Relationships		Do less of, or stop: Do more of, or start:
Drugs / Biology: Physical exercise, health, diet, sexual heath, alcohol, weight, smoking, caffeine etc		Do less of, or stop: Do more of, or start:

Practical Needs Assessment

Housing

- Does the patient have a place to live?
- Is it satisfactory?
- Does it place the patient at risk?
- Does the patient have a phone?
- Are there utilities in service?
- Is any type of housing assistance needed?

Employment
- What is the patient's employment status?
- Is this employment satisfactory?
- Is cocaine use a risk on the job?
- What services can be used to improve the situation?

Financial
- Is the patient in trouble financially?
- Is the patient in need of financial counseling?
- What financial services are needed?

Education
- Would the individual benefit from additional education?
- Is the patient interested in obtaining more education?
- re the patient's expectations realistic?

Health
- Does the patient have adequate health care?
- Is the patient or the family in need of health services?
- What health services could the patient use?

Legal
- Is the patient in need of legal assistance?
- What type of legal services would be helpful?

Childcare
- Does the patient need childcare services?
- What type of childcare would be helpful?

Transportation
- Does the patient need transportation services?
- What type of transportation would be helpful?

Areas of Concern, DSM IV Codes,

Associated Identifiers,

and

Long-term Goals

Anger

DSM IV Classification, Codes and Features: Conduct Disorder, NOS, 312.89
The essential feature of Conduct Disorder is a repetitive and persistent pattern in which the basic rights of others or major age-appropriate societal norms or rules are violated.

Associated Identifiers

1. Threatens or intimidates others
2. Initiates physical fights
3. Physically cruel to others
4. Physically cruel animals
5. Deliberately destroyed property
6. Lies to obtain goods and services
7. Stolen items
8. Often truant from work

Long –Term Goals

1. Participate in a recovery program that is free from addition and/or aggressive behavior.
2. Lower the incidence of angry thoughts, behavior and/or feelings.
3. Stop blaming others for your problems and accept personal responsibilities.
4. Obtain and maintain stress management skills

Antisocial Behavior

DSM IV Classification, Codes and Features: Antisocial Personality Disorder, 301.7
The essential features of Antisocial Personality Disorder is a pervasive pattern of disregard for, and violation of, the rights of others that begins in childhood or early adolescence and continues into adulthood.

Associated Identifiers
1. Failure to conform to social norms with respect to lawful behaviors
2. Deceitfulness, as indicated by repeated lying
3. Impulsivity or failure to plan ahead
4. Irritability/aggressiveness, as indicated by repeated physical fights or assaults
5. Reckless disregard for safety of self or others
6. Consistently blames others for own problems or behaviors
7. Lack of remorse having hurt, mistreated, or stolen from another
8. A history of many broken relationships

Long –Term Goals

1. Implement a program that is free from addition
2. Learn and implement new behaviors that are pro-social
3. Respect the rights and feelings of others
4. Abstain from addictive behaviors

Anxiety Disorder

DSM IV Classification, Codes and Features: Anxiety Disorder, 300.00
The essential feature of Generalized Anxiety Disorder is excessive anxiety and worry (apprehensive expectation), occurring more days than not for a period of at least 6 months, about a number of events or activities.

Associated Identifiers

1. Periods of accelerated heart beat
2. Periods of trembling or shaking
3. Sensations of shortness of breathe
4. Sensations of chest pain or discomfort
5. Periods of nausea or abdominal stress
6. Sensations of feeling dizzy or lightheaded
7. Periods of fear of losing control or dying
8. Periods of chills or hot flashes

Long –Term Goals

1. Stop addictive behavior as a means of escaping anxiety
2. Learn and understand the relationship between anxiety and addiction
3. Reduce anxious thoughts by increasing positive self-enhancing self-talk
4. Develop a social skills program to help reduce anxiety in social situations

Attention Deficit/Hyperactive Disorder

DSM IV Classification, Codes and Features: Attention Deficit/Hyperactive Disorder, 314.00

The essential feature of Attention-Deficit/Hyperactivity Disorder is a persistent pattern of inattention and/or hyperactivity-impulsivity that is more frequent and severe than is typically observed in individuals at a comparable level of development.

Associated Identifiers
1. Inattentive, easily distracted
2. Difficulty organizing thoughts
3. Easily distracted by noise or sights
4. Does not follow instructions
5. Forgets what he/she was doing
6. Gets caught up in the details and misses the big picture
7. Feeling apathetic or unmotivated
8. Lack clear goals or forward thinking
9. Short attention span
10. Finds it hard to keep mind on anything for very long

Long –Term Goals

1. Maintain a program of recovery from addiction and reduce the negative effects of ADHD
2. Develop necessary skills to understand and bring ADHD symptoms under control
3. Develop coping skills that are needed to improve ADHD symptoms and addiction
4. Understand the connection between addiction and ADHD behaviors

Inattention Symptom's
1. Trouble sustaining attention in routine situations (i.e., homework, chores, paperwork)
2. Avoids, dislikes, or is reluctant to engage in tasks that require sustained mental effort
3. Loses things
4. Lack clear goals or forward thinking
5. Difficulty expressing feelings
6. Difficulty expressing empathy for others
7. Excessive daydreaming
8. Feeling bored
9. Feeling apathetic or unmotivated
10. Feeling tired, sluggish or slow moving
11. Feeling spacey or "in a fog"

Impulse Control
1. Blows up at people in public.
2. Have angry outbursts that cannot control.
3. Gets into arguments and/or physical fights with people.
4. If angry with another driver, will tailgate that person or cut them off. (or if child) If angry with another person will take or break their belongings.
5. Often interrupts others.
6. Blurts out answers to questions before the questions have been completed.

7. Difficulty waiting in line or waiting my turn in games or group situations.
8. Feel a strong drive to be the "life of the party".
9. Feel a strong drive to be center stage in social settings.
10. Behaves or have behaved as the class "clown".
11. Says whatever thinking without regard to how it will affect others.
12. Make people feel uncomfortable when they are with me because they never know what will be said or done next.
13. Jumps from one activity or project to another activity or project without finishing any of them.

Borderline Personality Disorder

DSM IV Classification, Codes and Features: Borderline Personality Disorder,301.83
The essential feature of Borderline Personality Disorder is a pervasive pattern of instability of interpersonal relationships, self-image, and effects, and marked impulsivity that begins by early childhood and Is present in a variety of contexts.

Associated Identifiers

1. A pattern of unstable or intense interpersonal relationships
2. Unstable self-image or sense of self
3. Recurrent suicidal behavior, gestures, or threats
4. Chronic feelings of emptiness
5. Difficulty controlling anger
6. Feels unfairly treated
7. Feels others cannot be trusted
8. Impulsive behaviors that are potentially self-damaging

Long –Term Goals

1. Develop a program of recovery from addiction that reduces the impact of borderline traits on abstinence
2. Develop the ability to control impulses
3. Develop and demonstrate anger management skills
4. Reduce the frequency of self-damaging behaviors

Dependent Personality Disorder

DSM IV Classification, Codes and Features: Dependent Personality Disorder, 301.6
The essential feature of Dependent Personality Disorder is a pervasive and excessive need to be taken care of that leads to submissive and clinging behavior and fears of separations.

Associated Identifiers

1. Goes to excessive lengths to obtain nurturance and support
2. Feels uncomfortable or helpless when alone
3. Passively submissive to the wants and needs of others
4. Goes to excessively lengths to gain acceptance
5. Fearful of abandonment
6. Inability to trust own judgment
7. Persistent feelings of worthlessness
8. Chronic feelings of alienation from others

Long –Term Goals

1. Demonstrate increased independence and self-confidence
2. Decrease dependence on relationships
3. Demonstrate healthy communication that is honest
4. Improve feelings of self-worth by helping others in recovery

Depression

DSM IV Classification, Codes and Features: Disorder of: Depressive Disorder, NOS, 311
The Depressive Disorder Not Otherwise Specified category includes disorders with depressive features that do not meet the criteria for Major Depressive, Dysthymic or Adjustment.

Associated Identifiers

1. Cries easily
2. Feels alone
3. Feelings of worthlessness
4. Feels that I am a failure
5. Poor appetite
6. Low self-esteem
7. Have no appetite or over eats
8. Dislike myself
9. Do not enjoy activities that I used to enjoy
10. Tired all the time with no energy

Long –Term Goals

1. Elevate mood and develop a program of recovery that is free from addition
2. Decrease negative thinking and increase positive self-talk
3. Resolve interpersonal conflicts and grief issues
4. Increase feelings of self-worth and self-esteem

Expanded Questions (Depression)

1. Do not expect things to work out for me
2. Feel that I am a failure.
3. In situations where others appear to feel competent, I feel inadequate.
4. Have a harder time concentrating on work and other tasks than in the past.
5. Frequently think about dying or wishing were dead.
6. Either have a great deal of difficulty sleeping or sleep all the time.
7. Feel irritable and/or agitated
8. The future doesn't hold much interest for me.
9. Nothing in life is fun.
10. Blame self for many things.

Inability to Feel Positive Emotion

1. Difficulty understanding the concept of seeing the ``good" in a person or situation.
2. In the midst of situations in which other people are happy, I do not feel joy.
3. Watch, read or hear something that others find funny, but do not laugh.
4. In the midst of situations that others find exciting, do not feel exhilaration.

Dissociative Identity (Challenges)

DSM IV Classification, Codes and Features: Dissociative Disorder, NOS, 300.15
This category is included for disorders in which the predominate feature is dissociative symptoms (i.e., a disruption in the usual integrated functions of consciousness, memory, identity or perception of the environment) that does not meet the criteria for any specific Dissociative Disorder.

Associated Identifiers

1. Problem remembering events from childhood
2. Criticize self for all of my thoughts
3. Does not feel physical pain that most others do
4. Often hears voices inside my head
5. Often finds self in a setting but cannot recall how you got there
6. Often has out-of-body experiences
7. Do not like to look at self in mirror
8. Feel guilty all of the time
9. Cannot remember important personal events in life
10. Dislike self

Expanded Questions (Dissociative Disorder)

These questions are asked only if 40% or more of the screening questions are answered positively.

1. Find new things among my belongings that do not remember buying or receiving as a gift.
2. Often accused of lying when have not lied.
3. Sometimes remember past events so vividly that feel as if they are happening right now.

Emotional Disorder, Social
4. In situations where others do not feel shame, feel shame.
5. In situations where others do not feel guilt, feel guilt
6. Feel like whatever goes wrong is my fault.
7. Feel unacceptable.
8. Feel inadequate

Emotional Disorder, Primary
9. Am surprised at the elevated level of fear that surfaces in response to minor scares.
10. Am surprised at the elevated level of anger that surfaces in response to minor frustrations.
11. Am surprised at the elevated level of rage that surfaces in response to minor offenses.
12. Carry underlying fear.
13. Carry underlying anger.
14. Carry underlying rage.

Eating Disorder

DSM IV Classification, Codes and Features: Eating Disorder, NOS, 307.50
   The Eating Disorder, NOS category is for disorders of eating that may not meet the criteria for any specific Eating Disorder.

Associated Identifiers

1. Anxious when thinking about your body
2. Body image disturbance
3. Fear of becoming fat or gaining weight
4. Loss of control over eating
5. Intermittent starving, gorging, purging or using laxatives
6. Feelings of depression
7. Unable to bring abnormal eating habits under control
8. Uses food consumption as a means of relaxation and/or escape from stress

Long –Term Goals

1. Terminate overeating, purging, and use of laxatives
2. Develop healthy, realistic attitudes about body image and weight
3. Develop the ability to control impulses
4. Implement a program of addition recovery that reduces the impact of the eating disorder on sobriety

Expressive Language Disorder

DSM IV Classification, Codes and Features: Disorder of: Expressive Language Disorder, 315.31

The essential feature of Expressive Language Disorder is an impairment in expressive language development as demonstrated by scores on standardized individually administered measures of expressive language development substantially below those obtained from standardized measures of both nonverbal intellectual capacity and receptive language development.

Associated Identifiers

1. Speech is slow or labored
2. Uses immature grammar when speaking
3. Difficulty speaking spontaneously
4. Problems paraphrasing information presented orally
5. Uses incomplete, fragmented sentences
6. Difficulty expressing self in words
7. Problem finding the right word/words in conversation
8. Limited vocabulary
9. Problems organizing thoughts when speaking
10. Problems with speech/speaking causes problems at school/work

Expanded Questions (Speaking)

These questions are asked only if 40% or more of the screening questions are answered positively.

1. Cannot repeat sentences longer than 5 words.
2. Is slow to retrieve words.
3. Uses too many nonspecific nouns (e.g. thing, stuff) and indefinite   pronouns (e.g. that, there)
4. Uses too short or incomplete uttererances. (e.e. "You do")
5. Miss sequences phonemes when speaking (e.g. "aminals" for "animals")
6. Does not recall common word sequences (e.g. phone numbers, addresses).
7. Cannot say common blends (e.g. /bl/cr/fl/)
8. Cannot repeat words and phrases verbatim.
9. Have difficulty providing oral commands.
10. Retrieves the wrong words (e.g. asks for a crayon when wanting a pencil)
11. Have trouble talking around a subject or getting to the point in conversations.
12. Inability to express myself in speech causes problems for me in school, work or everyday life.
13. When speaking, uses incomplete sentences with numerous grammatical errors.
14. Often struggles for words to express self.
15. Have trouble telling a story in a logical order.

Impulsivity

DSM IV Classification, Codes and Features: Impulsive-Control Disorder, NOS, 312.30
This category is for disorders of impulse control that do not meet the criteria for any specific Impulse-Control Disorder or for another mental disorder having features involving impulse control (eg. Substance Dependence).

Associated Identifiers

1. Sense of tension or arousal prior to impulsive act
2. Sense of pleasure or gratification following an impulsive act
3. Desires immediate gratification
4. Little control over impulsive behaviors
5. Pattern of addictive behavior
6. Tendency to act too quickly
7. Difficulty being patient
8. History of acting out in areas that may be self-damaging

Long –Term Goals

1. Reduce frequency of impulsive behavior
2. Reduce thoughts that trigger impulsive behavior
3. Learn to stop, look, listen, think, and plan before acting
4. Maintain a program that is free from impulsive and addictive behavior

Legal Issues

DSM IV Classification, Codes and Features: Disruptive Behavior Disorder, NOS, 312.9
This category is for disorders characterized by conduct or oppositional defiant behaviors that do not meet the criteria for Conduct Disorder or Obsessive Defiant Disorder.

Associated Identifiers

1. Actively defies or refuses to comply with authoritative figures
2. Unresolved legal problems exacerbates the recovery process
3. Court ordered treatment for addictive behavior
4. Chemical dependency resulting in arrests
5. Fear of the legal system adjudicating current problems
6. Fear the loss of freedom due to current legal charges
7. Legal issues pending
8. History of legal involvement

Long –Term Goals

1. Accept responsibility for legal issues without blaming others
2. Consult with legal authorities to make plans for adjudicating legal conflicts
3. Maintain abstinence from addictive behaviors to remain free of negative consequences
4. Maintain a program of recovery that is free from addictive behavior and legal conflicts

Language Disorder

DSM IV Classification, Codes and Features: Disorder of: Mixed Receptive-Expressive Language Disorder, 315.31

The essential feature of Mixed Receptive-Expressive language Disorder is an impairment in both receptive and expressive language development as demonstrated by scores on standardized individually administered measures of both receptive expressive language development that are substantially below those obtained from standardized measures of nonverbal intellectual capacity.

Associated Identifiers

1. Misunderstands simple spoken sentences or questions
2. Misunderstands spoken directions
3. Does not comprehend spoken language but reads without difficulty
4. Difficulty remembering multi-spoken commands
5. Asks repeatedly for directions
6. Does not fully understand the speech of others
7. Difficulty understanding sentences that are spoken rapidly
8. Confuses simple nouns (hears cat, but thinks dog)
9. Difficulty with syntax (Dog chased the cat. Is the same as: Cat was chased by the dog.)
10. Problems listening causes problems at school/work

Expanded Questions (Listening)

These questions are asked only if 40% or more of the screening questions are answered positively.

1. Difficulty discriminating among speech sounds.
2. Difficulty understanding the meaning of long (i.e. multisyllabic) words.
3. Trouble understanding sentences that are spoken at a rapid rate, yet can understand them when they are spoken slowly.
4. Difficulty recognizing that two words begin or end with the same sound.
5. Difficulty recognizing that two words begin or end with a different sound.
6. Difficulty recognizing that two words contain the same or different sounds.
7. Difficulty with the nonliteral language (i.e. metaphors)

Language\Listening, Perception
16. When people are speaking can hear words, but the words are jumbled.
17. When listening to a conversation, realizes missing words.

Learning Disability--Sound\Voice (intonation, prosody but not words)
18. Able to hear sounds but the sounds are all jumbled.
19. Able to hear voices but the voices sound jumbled.
20. Difficulty separating voices from background noise.

Language\Listening

(Although I can hear words clearly)

21. Trouble hearing the differences between words.
22. Trouble accurately repeating what is said to me.

Language\Listening, Comprehension

(Although I can distinguish the differences between the sounds of words clearly)

23. Difficulty following spoken instructions.
24. Difficulty comprehending discussions in class, at work or with friends.
25. Misunderstands what people say.
26. Have difficulty comprehending what is said during telephone conversations.

Learning Disability--Sound\Voice (intonation, prosody but not words) Comprehension (Although I can hear the sound/voice clearly)

27. Have difficulty distinguishing the differences between voices.
28. Have difficulty hearing the rise and fall of pitch in voices; hear sound/voice as monotone.

Learning Disability--Sound\Voice (intonation, prosody but not words) Perception (Although I can hear the rise and fall in pitch of sound/voice clearly)

29. Difficulty understanding sarcasm.
30. Difficulty judging a person's mood by hearing their voice.
31. Difficulty knowing when someone is kidding or serious.
32. Difficulty knowing if someone is upset with me.
33. Difficulty knowing if a person is happy by hearing their voice.
34. Difficulty knowing if a person is sad by hearing their voice.

Living Arrangement

DSM IV Classification, Codes and Features: Relational Problems, NOS, V62.81
Relational problems include patterns of interaction between and among members of a relational unit that are associated with clinical significant impairment in functioning.

Associated Identifiers

1. Friends or relatives practice addictive behavior
2. Family angry with client and not supportive
3. Financially destitute and needs assistance
4. Peer group practices addictive behavior
5. Living environment has a high incidence of addictive behavior
6. Living environment poses a high risk for relapse
7. Socially isolated
8. Lives with individuals that practice addictive behavior

Long –Term Goals

1. Develop a peer group that is supportive of recovery
2. Improve social, occupational, financial, and living situation
3. Understand the negative impact that the current living situation has on recovery
4. Terminate addictive behaviors and implement more healthy coping behaviors to deal with family conflicts

Mathematics (Challenges)

DSM IV Classification, Codes and Features: Disorder of: Mathematics Disorder, 315.1
The essential feature of Mathematics Disorder is mathematical ability (as measured by individually administered standardized tests of mathematical calculation or reasoning) that falls substantially below that expected given the individual's chronological age, measured intelligence and age-appropriate education.

Associated Identifiers

1. Does not remember number words or digits
2. Makes mistakes when copying numbers
3. Reverses or transposes numbers
4. Problems counting a large number of objects
5. Reaches unreasonable conclusions when calculating mathematical problems
6. Cannot recall number facts automatically
7. Counts on fingers
8. Difficulty with multi-step mathematical problems
9. Difficulty with mathematical word problems
10. Mathematical problems causes problems at school/work

Expanded Questions (Mathematics)

These questions are asked only if 40% or more of the screening questions are answered positively.

1. Orders and spaces numbers inaccurately in multiplication and division
2. Misplaces digits in multi-digit numbers
3. Makes "borrowing" (i.e. regrouping/renaming)errors.
4. Disregards decimals
5. Reaches "unreasonable" answers.
6. Fails to verify answers and settles for first answers
7. Calculates poorly when the order of digit presentations is altered
8. Difficulty with the language of math
9. When looking at a math problem, does not know whether to add or subtract.
10. Makes math mistakes, like forgetting to carry numbers.
11. Add when meant to subtract.
12. When looking at a math equation, have a hard time knowing how to solve it.
13. Starts a math problem, but can't finish it because loses track of the steps halfway through.

Medical Issues

DSM IV Classification, Codes and Features: Psychological Symptoms Affecting Axis III (Medical), 316

> The essential feature of Psychological Factors Affecting Medical Condition is the presence of one or more specific psychological or behavioral factors that adversely affect a general medical condition.

Associated Identifiers

1. Medical issues impede recovery
2. Current medical issues lead to addictive behavior
3. Use of mood altering chemicals lead to self medicate problems
4. Use of mood altering chemicals has resulted in organic brain syndrome
5. Chronic pain places self at risk for relapse
6. Biomedical problems require medical assistance
7. Negative emotions surrounding medical issues has lead to addictive behavior
8. Incapable of self administering of prescribed medication

Long –Term Goals

1. Resolve current medical issues
2. Understand relationship between addictive behaviors and medical issues
3. Reduce impact of medical issues on recovery
4. Maintain a recovery program that is free from addiction and the negative effects of medical issues

Memory Challenges

DSM IV Classification, Codes and Features: Disorder of: Cognitive Disorder, NOS, 294.9
This category is for disorders that are characterized by cognitive dysfunction presumed to be due to the direct physiological effect of a general medical condition that do not meet criteria for any of the specific deliriums, dementias or amnestic disorders listed.

Associated Identifiers

1. Remembers things from the past but not recent events
2. Cannot remember events from one day to the next
3. Difficulty following two or more step directions
4. Does not follow through on instructions
5. Forgets want he/she was doing.
6. Difficulties engaging in tasks
7. When given 3 things to do, remembers only the first or last
8. Trouble with chores or tasks requiring more than one step
9. When shopping, I must make a list or I'll forget items needed
10. Problems with my memory causes problems at school/work

Expanded Questions (Memory Challenges)

These questions are asked only if 40% or more of the screening questions are answered positively.

Memory
1. Fails to finish schoolwork, chores and/or workplace duties.
2. Problems remembering things even for one minute.
3. Trouble following directions that have more than one or two steps.

Memory Dysfunction--Visual, Spatial\Facial
4. Have an inability to remember faces.
5. Can't remember features of where he/she used to live or work.
6. Can't remember what my childhood neighborhood looked like.
7. Trouble remembering where things are located in my house.
8. When trying to give directions to someone can't remember the sequence of landmarks or turns.
9. Trouble remembering where things were put.
10. When going out, have trouble remembering where car is parked.
11.. Cannot remember features of a painting, photograph or map immediately after finished viewing it.
12. When it is dark or with eyes closed, have difficulty walking through my house.
13. Memory Dysfunction--Auditory, Sound\Voice (intonation, prosody but not words)
14. Difficulty remembering what a person's voice sounded like if after talking to them for the first time earlier that day.

15. Have difficulty remembering what a person's voice sounds like if after knowing them for a long time.
16. When listening to a singer, have difficulty remembering his voice to match it to other songs that he sings.

Memory Dysfunction--Auditory, Language\Listening
17. If someone tells me their address, phone number or e-mail address, he/she forgets it unless written down.
18. Have difficulty recalling the name of someone just met.
19. When asked to pick up two or three items at the store, must have a written list or forgets.
20. Have difficulty recalling the names of people that have known for a long time.

Obsessive-Compulsive Disorder

DSM IV Classification, Codes and Features: Disorder of: Obsessive-Compulsive Disorder, 300.3

The essential features of Obsessive-Compulsive Disorder are recurrent obsessions or compulsions that are severe enough to be time consuming (i.e., they take more than 1 hour a day) or cause marked distress or significant impairment.

Associated Identifiers

1. Inability to deviate from the routine
2. Greater need than others to keep things in order
3. Must control people and situations
4. Driven to perform a behavior over and over again
5. Inability to alter unproductive/destructive behaviors
6. Work/school is far more important than friends
7. Preoccupied with rules, lists and/or details
8. Ideas/feelings play over and over again, like a broken record
9. Stubborn
10. Preoccupied with feelings that something bad may happen

Expanded Questions (Obsessive-Compulsive Disorder)

These questions are asked only if 40% or more of the screening questions are answered positively.

1. Focus so much on doing tasks perfectly that I fail to complete them.
2. Working or schoolwork is far more important to me than having friends.
3. Reluctant to delegate work to others unless they submit to my way of doing things.
4. Feel driven to perform a behavior over and over again, such as hand washing, counting or repeating a word to myself.
5. Have to check again and again whether I have done something, such as turning off an appliance or locking a door.
6. Have to do things very slowly to make absolutely sure they are done correctly.

Thoughts:

7. Have thoughts that I don't like, but I can't stop thinking them.
8. Worry about things that are not real-life problems.
9. Have the feeling that something bad will happen if I don't do certain behaviors even though I know that there is no connection

Occupational Problems

DSM IV Classification, Codes and Features: Occupational Problems, V62.2
This category can be used when the focus of clinical attention is an occupational problem that is not due in part to a mental disorder.

Associated Identifiers

1. Stressful work environment lead to addictive behaviors
2. Coworkers use illegal drugs and alcohol
3. Employer does not understand the recovery process
4. Job in jeopardy due to addictive behavior
5. Unemployed due to addictive behaviors
6. Feelings of inadequacy at the work place inhibits addictive behaviors
7. Addictive behavior due to retirement
8. Conflicts with authority figures lead to addictive behavior

Long –Term Goals

1. Contract with management team that details a recovery plan
2. Communicate and gain support from peers to help recovery
3. Fill life with new interest
4. Maintain a recovery program that is free from addiction and occupational issues

Oppositional Defiant (Challenges)

DSM IV Classification, Codes and Features: Disorder of: Oppositional Defiant Disorder, 313.81

The essential feature of Oppositional Defiant Disorder is a recurrent pattern of negativistic, defiant, disobedient and hostile behavior toward authority figures that persists for at least 6 months. To qualify for Oppositional Defiant Disorder, behaviors must occur more frequently than is typically observed in individuals of comparable age and development level and must lead to significant impairment in social, academic or occupational functioning.

Associated Identifiers
1. Often disobeys the rules
2. Argues with others
3. Argues
4. Deliberately annoys others
5. Often looses temper
6. Often angry and resentful
7. Irritable
8. Spiteful and vindictive
9. Inability to feel negative emotions
10. Intentionally disregards socially acceptable behavior

Long –Term Goals

1. Maintain a recovery program that is free from addiction and oppositional defiant behaviors
2. Follow family rules without confrontation
3. Learn new coping skills
4. Learn assertiveness skills that are necessary to reduce anger

Expanded Questions (Oppositional-Defiant Disorder)

These questions are asked only if 40% or more of the screening questions are answered positively.

1. Small events trigger big reactions
2. Gets into trouble if not closely supervised
3. Angry outburst are intense but end suddenly
4. Touchy or easily annoyed by others.
5. Hard to control in public settings

Elevated Anger, Rage, Fear
6. In the midst of situations that others find frightening, feelings of fear seem less intense than those of others around me.
7. When someone seriously wrongs or insults me, sense less anger than others seem to feel.
8. In the midst of unfair and unjust situations in which others express anger and rage, feelings of anger and rage seem less intense.

9. In the midst of unfair and unjust situations observed happening to others (through reading, movies, etc.), feel less anger or rage than others seem to feel.
10. In the midst of situations in which others feel anxious, feelings of anxiety seem less intense than those of others around me.
11. Inability to Feel Negative Emotion
12. In situations where most people would not feel fear, feel afraid.
13. In situations where most people would not feel anger, feel angry.
14. In situations where most people would feel angry, feel enraged.
15. Angered by people's stupidity.
16. When a person cuts in front of me while driving, feel enraged.
17. Have urges to break or smash things.
18. Feel intense anger over insignificant things.
19. Have to avoid things, places or activities that most people seem relatively comfortable with because they frighten me.

Partner Relationship Problems

DSM IV Classification, Codes and Features: Partner Relationship Disorder, V61.1
This category is used when the focus of clinical attention is a pattern of interaction between spouses or partners characterized by negative communication, distorted communication, or non-communication that is associated with clinically significant impairment in individual or family functioning or the development of symptoms in one or both partners.

Associated Identifiers

1. Inability to establish and maintain meaningful relationships
2. Pattern of abuse leading to addictive behaviors
3. Emotional disturbance from partner
4. Pending divorce
5. Lack of communication with significant other
6. Pattern of addictive behavior leading to social isolation
7. Verbally abusive or physical abusive relationship
8. Involvement in multiple superficial relationships

Long –Term Goals

1. Terminate addictive behavior and resolve relationship conflicts
2. Decrease partner relational conflicts
3. Develop skills needed to maintain open and effective relationships
4. Maintain a recovery program that is free from addiction and partner relational conflicts

Posttraumatic Stress Disorder

DSM IV Classification, Codes and Features: Posttraumatic Stress Disorder, 309.81
The essential feature of Posttraumatic Stress Disorder is the development of characteristic symptoms following exposure to an extreme traumatic stressor involving personal experience of an event that involves actual or threatened death or serious injury.

Associated Identifiers

1. Feelings as if a traumatic event is again recurring
2. Recurrent intrusive memories of a traumatic event
3. Inability to recall parts of a traumatic experience
4. Recurring thoughts of a traumatic event causes addictive behavior
5. Feeling of detachment
6. difficulty falling or staying asleep
7. Engaging in addictive behavior to escape traumatic event
8. Avoids feelings, thoughts, or conversations about the traumatic event

Long –Term Goals

1. Resolve emotional effects of past traumas
2. Learn and demonstrate new coping skills
3. Understand posttraumatic stress symptoms and how they led to addictive behaviors
4. Maintain a recovery program that is free from addiction and posttraumatic stress symptoms

A. The person has been exposed to a traumatic event in which both of the following were present:

(1) the person experienced, witnessed, or was confronted with an event or events that involved actual or threatened death or serious injury, or a threat to the physical integrity of self or others

(2) the person's response involved intense fear, helplessness, or horror. Note: In children, this may be expressed instead by disorganized or agitated behavior

B. The traumatic event is persistently re-experienced in one (or more) of the following ways:

(1) recurrent and intrusive distressing recollections of the event, including images, thoughts, or perceptions. Note: In young children, repetitive play may occur in which themes or aspects of the trauma are expressed.

(2) recurrent distressing dreams of the event. Note: In children, there may be frightening dreams without recognizable content.

(3) acting or feeling as if the traumatic event were recurring (includes a sense of reliving the experience, illusions, hallucinations, and dissociative flashback episodes, including those that occur on awakening or when intoxicated). Note: In young children, trauma-specific reenactment may occur.

(4) intense psychological distress at exposure to internal or external cues that symbolize or resemble an aspect of the traumatic event

(5) physiological reactivity on exposure to internal or external cues that symbolize or resemble an aspect of the traumatic event

C. Persistent avoidance of stimuli associated with the trauma and numbing of general responsiveness (not present before the trauma), as indicated by three (or more) of the following:

(1) efforts to avoid thoughts, feelings, or conversations associated with the trauma
(2) efforts to avoid activities, places, or people that arouse recollections of the trauma
(3) inability to recall an important aspect of the trauma
(4) markedly diminished interest or participation in significant activities
(5) feeling of detachment or estrangement from others
(6) restricted range of affect (e.g., unable to have loving feelings)
(7) sense of a foreshortened future (e.g., does not expect to have a career, marriage, children, or a normal life span)

D. Persistent symptoms of increased arousal (not present before the trauma), as indicated by two (or more) of the following:

(1) difficulty falling or staying asleep
(2) irritability or outbursts of anger
(3) difficulty concentrating
(4) hyper-vigilance
(5) exaggerated startle response

E. Duration of the disturbance (symptoms in Criteria B, C, and D) is more than 1 month.

F. The disturbance causes clinically significant distress or impairment in social, occupational, or other important areas of functioning.

Specify if:
Acute: if duration of symptoms is less than 3 months
Chronic: if duration of symptoms is 3 months or more

Specify if:
With Delayed Onset: if onset of symptoms is at least 6 months after the stressor

A. The person has been exposed to a traumatic event in which both of the following were present:
(1) the person experienced, witnessed, or was confronted with an event or events that involved actual or threatened death or serious injury, or a threat to the physical integrity of self or others

(2) the person's response involved intense fear, helplessness, or horror. Note: In children, this may be expressed instead by disorganized or agitated behavior

B. The traumatic event is persistently re-experienced in one (or more) of the following ways:

(1) recurrent and intrusive distressing recollections of the event, including images, thoughts, or perceptions. Note: In young children, repetitive play may occur in which themes or aspects of the trauma are expressed.

(2) recurrent distressing dreams of the event. Note: In children, there may be frightening dreams without recognizable content.

(3) acting or feeling as if the traumatic event were recurring (includes a sense of reliving the experience, illusions, hallucinations, and dissociative flashback episodes, including those that occur on awakening or when intoxicated). Note: In young children, trauma-specific reenactment may occur.

(4) intense psychological distress at exposure to internal or external cues that symbolize or resemble an aspect of the traumatic event

(5) physiological reactivity on exposure to internal or external cues that symbolize or resemble an aspect of the traumatic event
C. Persistent avoidance of stimuli associated with the trauma and numbing of general responsiveness (not present before the trauma), as indicated by three (or more) of the following:

(1) efforts to avoid thoughts, feelings, or conversations associated with the trauma
(2) efforts to avoid activities, places, or people that arouse recollections of the trauma
(3) inability to recall an important aspect of the trauma
(4) markedly diminished interest or participation in significant activities
(5) feeling of detachment or estrangement from others
(6) restricted range of affect (e.g., unable to have loving feelings)
(7) sense of a foreshortened future (e.g., does not expect to have a career, marriage, children, or a normal life span)

D. Persistent symptoms of increased arousal (not present before the trauma), as indicated by two (or more) of the following:

(1) difficulty falling or staying asleep
(2) irritability or outbursts of anger
(3) difficulty concentrating
(4) hyper-vigilance
(5) exaggerated startle response

E. Duration of the disturbance (symptoms in Criteria B, C, and D) is more than 1 month.

F. The disturbance causes clinically significant distress or impairment in social, occupational, or other important areas of functioning.

Specify if:
Acute: if duration of symptoms is less than 3 months
Chronic: if duration of symptoms is 3 months or more
Specify if:
With Delayed Onset: if onset of symptoms is at least 6 months after the stressor

Reading (Challenges)

DSM IV Classification, Codes and Features: Reading Disorder, 315.00
The essential feature of Reading Disorder is reading achievement (i.e., reading accuracy, speed, or comprehension as measured by individually administered standardized tests) that falls substantially below that expected given the individual's chronological age, measured intelligence and age-appropriate education.

Associated Identifiers

1. Limited sight vocabulary
2. Cannot sound out words
3. Does not like to read
4. Slow silent reader
5. Skips words when reading aloud
6. Reads the same line twice
7. Cannot retell what has been read
8. Eyes hurt and/or water while reading
9. Difficulty understanding the main idea or identifying important details from a story
10. Difficulty with reading causes problems at school/work

Expanded Questions (Reading)

These questions are asked only if 40% or more of the screening questions are answered positively.

P=Perception   *C=Comprehension*
V=Visual   *E=Expressive*

Areas of Concern: Reading

1. Poor memory for letters and words
2. Slow oral reader.
3. Substitutes phonetically similar words while reading aloud (e.g. "chair" for cheer "then" for when) P
4. Interchanges little words, especially articles ("a" for "the") when reading orally. P
5. Reverses letters in oral reading (e.g. b as d) P
6. Makes errors when reading unfamiliar words aloud
7. Confuses words that appear similar (e.g. "bread" for broad) P
8. Omits inflectional endings (i.e. –s,-ed,-ing) when reading aloud
9. Cannot break a word into words
10. Cannot combine syllables into words
11. Cannot call non words
12. Has problems remembering what is read even though I have read all the words. C
13. Switches letters in words when reading (such as god and dog).
14. Words tend to blur while reading.

15. Words tend to move around the page when reading.
16. When reading aloud, substitutes words.
17. Words don't make sense to me when reading them.
18. Read a paragraph, but cannot tell you what has been read. C
19. Have difficulty comprehending/understanding what is read even if reread. C
20. Have difficulty remembering addresses seen. V
21. Have difficulty remembering phone numbers seen. V
22. Have difficulty remembering my social security number. C
23. Have difficulty remembering quotes after read. C
24. Difficulty with reading causes problems for me in school, work, or everyday life.

Social Phobia

DSM IV Classification, Codes and Features: Social Phobia, 300.23
The essential feature **DSM** of Social Phobia is a marked and persistent fear of social or performance situations in which embarrassment may occur. Exposure to the social or performance situation almost invariably provokes an immediate anxiety response.

Associated Identifiers

1. Often feels no shame
2. Often feels no guilt
3. Often feels inadequate
4. Often feels unaccepted
5. Feels as if everything that goes wrong is your fault
6. Minor surprises are often elevated to high levels of fear
7. Minor frustrations are often elevated to high levels of fear
8. Underlying fear is always present
9. Underlying anger is always present
10. Underlying rage is always present

Long –Term Goals

1. Interact socially without excessive anxiety
2. Develop social skills that are necessary to reduce stress
3. Decrease thoughts that trigger anxiety
4. Form relationships that will enhance a support system

Expanded Questions (Social/Primary)

These questions are asked only if 40% or more of the screening questions are answered positively.

Comprehending Social Cues Dysfunction

1. Have difficulty knowing how people feel about me unless they put it into words.
2. Do not understand why people laugh when they do.
3. Have difficulty distinguishing when a person is joking or serious.
4. Have difficulty understanding when a person is being sarcastic.
5. Have difficulty discerning when a person is upset with me.
6. Difficulty predicting a person's reactions
7. Difficulty resolving personal conflicts
8. Difficulty using/understanding relevant language in social context
9. Often offends or annoys others when they speak
10. Difficulty obtaining respect/admiration of others

Substance Abuse Challenges

DSM IV Classification, Codes, and Features: Substance Abuse (Other), 305.90
The essential feature of Substance Abuse is a maladaptive pattern of substance use manifested by recurrent and significant adverse consequences related to the repeated use of substances. These problems must occur recurrently during the same 12-month period.

Associated Identifiers

1. Have you used drugs other than those required for medical reasons?	Yes	No
2. Have you abused prescription drugs?	Yes	No
3. Do you abuse more than one drug at a time?	Yes	No
4. Can you get through the week without using drugs (other than those required for medical reasons)?	Yes	No
5. Are you always able to stop using drugs when you want to?	Yes	No
6. Do you abuse drugs on a continuous basis?	Yes	No
7. Do you try to limit your drug use to certain situations?	Yes	No
8. Have you had "blackouts" or "flashbacks" as a result of drug use?	Yes	No
9. Do you ever feel bad about your drug abuse?	Yes	No
10. Does your spouse (or parents) ever complain about your involvement with drugs?	Yes	No

Long –Term Goals

1. Withdraw from mood altering substances and establish a supportive recovery plan
2. Establish a sustained recovery program
3. Establish and maintain total abstinence
4. accept own chemical dependence and begin to actively participate in a recovery program

Expanded Questions (Substance Abuse)

These questions are asked only if 40% or more of the screening questions are answered positively.

1. Do friends or relatives know or suspect you abuse drugs?	Yes	No
2. Have drug abuse ever created problems between you and your spouse?	Yes	No
3. Have any family member ever sought help for problems related to your drug use?	Yes	No
4. Have you ever lost friends because of your use of drugs?	Yes	No
5. Have you ever neglected your family or missed work because of your use of drugs?	Yes	No
6. Have you ever been in trouble at work because of drug abuse?	Yes	No
7. Have you ever lost a job because of drug abuse?	Yes	No
8. Have you gotten into fights when under the influence of drugs?	Yes	No

9. Have you ever been arrested because of unusual behavior while under the influence of drugs?   Yes   No

10. Have you ever been arrested for driving while under the influence of drugs?   Yes   No

11. Have you engaged in illegal activities to obtain drugs?   Yes   No

12. Have you ever been arrested for possession of illegal drugs?   Yes   No

13. Have you ever experienced withdrawal symptoms as a result of heavy drug intake?   Yes   No

14. Have you had medical problems as a result of your drug use (e.g., memory loss, hepatitis, convulsions, or bleeding)?   Yes   No

15. Have you ever gone to anyone for help for a drug problem?   Yes   No

16. Have you ever been in hospital for medical problems related to your drug use?   Yes   No

17. Have you ever been involved in a treatment program specifically related to drug use?   Yes   No

18. Have you been treated as an outpatient for problems related to drug abuse?   Yes   No

Suicidal Ideation

DSM IV Classification, Codes and Features: Substance-Induced Mood Disorder, Other, 292.84

The essential feature of Substance-Induced Mood Disorder is a prominent and persistent Disturbance of mood that is judged to be due to the direct physiological effects of a substance.

Associated Identifiers

1. Elevated or irritable mood
2. Depressed mood
3. Diminished interest in all or almost all activities
4. Ongoing suicidal ideation with a specific plan
5. Ongoing suicidal ideation without a specific plan
6. Personal loses due to addictive behavior
7. History of suicide attempts
8. Addictive behavior exacerbates depression, hopelessness and/or suicidal ideation

Long –Term Goals

1. Resolve the wish for death and find new hope
2. Terminate all suicide urges
3. Understand the relationship between suicidal ideation and addictive behaviors
4. Enter a level of care program that is necessary to protect self from suicidal impulses

Writing (Challenges)

DSM IV Classification, Codes and Features: Disorder of Written Expression, 315.2

The essential feature of Disorder of Written Expression Reading is writing skills (as measured by individually administered standardized tests or functional assessment of writing skills) that falls substantially below that expected given the individual's chronological age, measured intelligence and age-appropriate education.

Associated Identifiers

1. Reverses letters of words
2. Adds unnecessary letters when spelling words
3. Handwriting is messy
4. Problems with grammar and/or punctuation
5. Problems copying off the board or from print
6. Problems getting thoughts on paper when writing
7. Can retell a story but cannot write it
8. Difficulty expressing self when writing
9. Problems organizing thoughts into paragraphs when writing
10. Difficulty writing causes problems at school/work

Expanded Questions (Writing)

These questions are asked only if 40% or more of the screening questions are answered positively.

1. Miss spells irregular words by attempting to spell phonetically
2. Writes with limited output (e.g. essays too short, few words and sentences)
3. Omits words in sentences
4. Omits endings in words
5. Misspells words so badly that no one has any idea what they are
6. Omits letters when spelling
7. Spell words with the correct letters but in the wrong sequences (htnig for thing)
8. Writes sentence fragments
9. Does not write complex sentences (i.e. consistently writes short, simple sentences)
10. Work tends to be messy.
11. Prefers print rather than writing in cursive.
12. Letters run into each other or there is no space between words.
13. Have trouble staying within lines.
14. Makes grammar and punctuation mistakes when writing.
15. When writing, have trouble recalling the right letters or words.

1. Light sensitive. Bothered by glare, sunlight, headlights or streetlights.
2. Becomes tired, experience headaches, feels restless or has an inability to stay focused with bright or fluorescent lights.
3. When reading words or letters shift, shake, blur, move, run together, disappear or become difficult to perceive.

Learning Disability--Spatial\Facial
(Although my eyesight is normal.)
  4. When looking at a picture or object it seem clear.
  5. When looking at a picture or object only sees part of it.

Learning Disability--Spatial\Facial, Perception
  6. Difficulty telling people apart if they have similar features, such as the same color hair.

Learning Disability--Spatial\Facial, Comprehension
  7. Difficulty knowing east from west and north from south.
  8. When looking at a picture have difficulty identifying the images it contains.
  9. When looking at a person's face have difficulty knowing if they are upset.
  10. When looking at a person's face have difficulty knowing if they are sad.
  11. When looking at a person's face have difficulty knowing if they are happy.
  12. When looking at a person's face have difficulty knowing if they are upset with me.
  13. When looking at a person's face have difficulty knowing if they are joking or serious.

Body Awareness/ Spatial Relationships
  1. Trouble with knowing my left from my right.
  2. Difficulty with concepts such as up, down, over or under.
  3. Neuro-sensory Integration Disorder

Right
  4. Difficulty catching balls.
  5. Difficulty skipping rope
  6. Difficulty knowing which way to move if someone yells "Get out of way!"
  7. Trouble putting together Lego's or Lincoln logs. Has difficulty putting together puzzles

Left
  8. When given assignments orally I have difficulty copying them into my assignment book.

Sensory Integration Issues
  9. Seem to be more sensitive to the environment than others.
  10. Unusual sensitivity to certain smells.
  11. Unusual sensitivity to light.
  12. Sensitive to movement or craves spinning activities?
  13. Tend to be clumsy or accident prone.

Learning Disability--Somato-sensory, Perception
  14. When eyes closed my eyes, have difficulty touching my finger to my nose.
  15. Difficulty knowing which way to move if someone yells "Get out of the way!"
  16. Difficulty sensing the position of my body without looking at it.
  17. When touched, have little awareness of it.

Alternative

Screening

Tools

Conner's' Behavior Rating Scale

1. Inattentive, easily distracted... 0   1   2   3

2. Angry and resentful.. 0   1   2   3

3. Difficulty doing or completing homework/chores/tasks..................0   1   2   3

4. Is always "on the go"...0   1   2   3

5. Short attention span..0   1   2   3

6. Argues with adults..0   1   2   3

7. Fidgets with hands or feet or squirms in seat.............................0   1   2   3

8. Fails to complete assigns/chores/tasks....................................0   1   2   3

9. Hard to control in malls or while shopping...............................0   1   2   3

10. Messy or disorganized at school, home, work............................0   1   2   3

11. Loses temper..0   1   2   3

12. Needs close supervision to get through chores, assignments, tasks.......0   1   2   3

13. Only attends if it is something he/she is very interested in................0   1   2   3

14. Runs about/climbs excessively where it is inappropriate….................0   1   2   3

15. Distractibility or attention span a problem...............................0   1   2   3

16. Irritable..0   1   2   3

17. Avoids, expresses reluctance about, or has difficulties engaging in
tasks that requires sustained mental effort (work/schoolwork)...........0   1   2   3

18. Restless in the "squirmy sense"...0   1   2   3

19. Gets distracted when giving instructions to do something.................0   1   2   3

20. Actively distracted when given instructions to do something.............0   1   2   3

21. Has trouble concentrating in class..0   1   2   3

22. Has difficulty waiting in lines or waiting turn in games or
group situations…. 0   1   2   3

23. Leaves seat in classroom or in other situations in which
remaining seated   is expected...0   1   2   3

24. Deliberately does things that annoy other people..........................0   1   2   3

25. Does not follow through on instructions and fails to finish work.........0   1   2   3

26. Has difficulty playing or engaging in leisure activities quietly...........0   1   2   3

27. Easily frustrated in efforts...,,,0   1   2   3

Behavior Rating Inventory of Executive Functioning

1. Overreacts to small problems.	N	S	O
2. When given three things to do, remembers only the last.	N	S	O
3. Is not a self starter.	N	S	O
4. Cannot get a disappointment, scolding or insult off his/her mind.	N	S	O
5. Resists or has trouble accepting a different way to solve a problem with schoolwork, friends, chores, etc.	N	S	O
6. Becomes upset with new situations.	N	S	O
7. Has explosive, angry outbursts.	N	S	O
8. Has short attention span.	N	S	O
9. Needs to be told "no" or "stop that".	N	S	O
10. Needs to be told to begin a task even when willing.	N	S	O
11. Loses lunch box, lunch money, permission slips, homework, etc	N	S	O
12. Does not bring home homework, assignment sheets, material, etc.	N	S	O
13. Acts upset by change in plans.	N	S	O
14. Is disrupted by change of teacher or class.	N	S	O
15. Does not check work for mistakes.	N	S	O
16. Cannot find clothes, glasses, shoes, toys, books, pencils, etc.	N	S	O
17. Has good ideas but cannot get them on paper.	N	S	O
18. Has trouble concentrating on chores, schoolwork, etc	N	S	O
19. Does not show creativity in solving a problem.	N	S	O
20. Backpack is disorganized.	N	S	O
21. Is easily distracted by, noises, activity, sights, etc.	N	S	O
22. Makes careless errors.	N	S	O
23. Forgets to hand in homework, even when completed.	N	S	O
24. Resists change to routine, foods, places, etc.	N	S	O
25. Has trouble with chores or tasks	N	S	O
26. Has outbursts for little reason.	N	S	O
27. Mood changes frequently.	N	S	O
28. Needs help from adult to stay at task.	N	S	O
29. Gets caught up in details and misses the big picture.	N	S	O
30. has trouble getting used to new situations (classes, groups, friend's)	N	S	O
31. Forgets what he/she is doing.	N	S	O
32. When sent to get something, forgets what he/she is supposed to get.	N	S	O
33. Is unaware of how his/her behavior affects or bothers others.	N	S	O
34. Has problems coming up with different ways to solve a problem.	N	S	O
35. Has good ideas but does not get job done (lacks follow-though)	N	S	O
36. Leaves work incomplete.	N	S	O
37. Becomes overwhelmed by large assignments.	N	S	O
38. Does not think before doing.	N	S	O
39. Has trouble finishing tasks.	N	S	O
40. Thinks too much about the same topic.	N	S	O
41. Underestimates time needed to finish tasks.	N	S	O
42. Interrupts others	N	S	O

Behavior Rating Inventory of Executive Functioning

43. Is impulsive.	N	S	O
44. Does not notice when his/her behavior causes negative reactions.	N	S	O
45. Gets out of seat at the wrong times.	N	S	O
46. Is Unaware of own behavior when in a group.	N	S	O
47. Gets out of control more than friends.	N	S	O
48. Reacts more strongly to situations than other children.	N	S	O
49. Starts assignments or chores at the last minute.	N	S	O
50. Has trouble getting started on homework or chores.	N	S	O
51. Mood is easily influenced by the situation.	N	S	O
52. Does not plan ahead for school assignments	N	S	O
53. Gets stuck on one topic or activity.	N	S	O
54. Has poor understanding of own strengths and weaknesses.	N	S	O
55. Talks or plays too loud.	N	S	O
56. Written work is poorly organized	N	S	O
57. Acts too wild or "out of control".	N	S	O
58. Has trouble putting the brakes on his/her actions.	N	S	O
59. Gets in trouble if not supervised by an adult.	N	S	O
60. Has trouble putting the brakes on his/her actions.	N	S	O
61. Work is sloppy.	N	S	O
62. After having a problem, will stay disappointed for a long time.	N	S	O
63. Does not take initiative.	N	S	O
64. Angry or tearful outbursts are intensive but end suddenly.	N	S	O
65. Does not realize that certain actions bother others.	N	S	O
66. Small events trigger big reactions.	N	S	O
67. Cannot find things in room or school desk.	N	S	O
68. Leaves a trail of belongings wherever he/she goes.	N	S	O
69. Does not think of consequences before acting.	N	S	O
70. Trouble thinking of a different way to solve a problem when stuck.	N	S	O
71. Leaves messes that others have to clean up.	N	S	O
72. Becomes upset to easily.	N	S	O
73. Has a messy desk.	N	S	O
74. Has trouble waiting for turn.	N	S	O
75. Does not connect doing tonight's homework with grades.	N	S	O
76. Tests poorly even when knows correct answers.	N	S	O
77. Does not finish long-term projects.	N	S	O
78. Has poor handwriting.	N	S	O
79. Has to be closely supervised.	N	S	O
80. Has trouble moving from one activity to another.	N	S	O
81. Is fidgety.	N	S	O
82. Cannot stay on the same topic when talking.	N	S	O
83. Blurts thinks out.	N	S	O
84. Says the same things over and over.	N	S	O
85. Talks at the wrong time.	N	S	O
86. Does not come prepared for class.	N	S	O

Beck's Depression Inventory-II (BDI-II)

1. **Sadness**
   - 0   I do not feel sad
   - 1 I feel sad much of the time
   - 2 I am sad all of the time
   - 3 I am so sad or unhappy that I can't stand it

2. **Pessimism**
   - 0. I am not discouraged about my future
   - 1. I feel more discouraged about my future than I used to be
   - 2. I do not expect things to work out for me
   - 3. I feel my future is hopeless and will only get worst

3. **Past Failure**
   - 0 I do not feel like a failure
   - 1 I have failed more than I should have
   - 2 As I look back, I see a lot of failures
   - 3 I feel I am a total failure as a person

4. **Loss of Pleasure**
   - 0 I get as much pleasure as I ever did from the things I enjoy
   - 1 I don't enjoy things as much as I used to
   - 2 I get very little pleasure from the things I used to enjoy
   - 3 I can't get any pleasure from the things I used to enjoy

5. **Guilty Feelings**
   - 4 I don't feel particularly guilty
   - 5 I feel guilty over many things that I have done or should have done
   - 6 I feel quiet guilty most of the time
   - 7 I feel guilty all of the time

6. **Punishment Feelings**
   - 8 I don't feel I am being punished
   - 9 I feel I am being punished
   - 10 I expect to be punished
   - 11 I feel I am being punished

7. **Self-Dislike**
   - 12 I feel the same about myself as ever
   - 13 I have lost confidence in myself
   - 14 I am disappointed in myself
   - 15 I dislike myself

8. Self-Criticalness
16 I don't criticize or blame myself more than usual
17 I am more critical of myself than I used to be
18 I criticize myself for all of my faults
19 I blame myself for everything bad that happens

9. Suicidal Thoughts or Wishes
20 I don't have any thoughts of killing myself
21 I have thoughts of killing myself, but I would not carry them out
22 I would like to kill myself
23 I would kill myself if I had the chance

10. Crying
24 I don't cry anymore than I used to
25 I cry more than I used to
26 I cry over every little thing
27 I feel like crying, but I can't

11. Agitation
28 I am no more restless or wound up than usual
29 I feel more restless and wound up than usual
30 I am so restless or agitated that it's hard to stay still
31 I am so restless or agitated that I have to keep moving or doing something

12. Loss of Interest
0 I have not lost interest in other people or activities
1 I am less interested in other people or things than before
2 I have lost most of my interest in other people or things
3 It's hard to get interested in anything

13. Indecisiveness
0 I make decisions about as well as ever
1 I find it more difficult to make decisions than usual
2 I have much greater difficulty in making decisions than I used to
3 I have trouble making any decisions

14. Worthlessness
0 I do not feel I am worthless
1 I don't consider myself as worthwhile and useful as I used to
2 I feel more worthless as compared to other people
3 I feel utterly worthless

15. Loss of Energy
0 I have as much energy as ever
1 I have less energy than I used to have
2 I don't have enough energy to do very much
3 I don't have enough energy to do anything

16. Changes in sleep

0   I have not experienced any change in my sleeping pattern
1a   I sleep somewhat more than I used to
1b   I sleep somewhat less than usual
2a   I sleep a lot more than usual
2b   I sleep a lot less than usual
3a   I sleep most of the day
3b   I wake up 1-2 hours early and can't get back to sleep

17. Irritability

0   I am no more irritable than usual
1   I am more irritable than usual
2   I am much more irritable than usual
3   I am irritable all the time

18. Changes in Appetite

0   I have not experienced any change in my appetite
1a   My appetite is somewhat less than usual
1b   My appetite is somewhat greater than usual
2a   My appetite is much less than before
2b   My appetite is much greater than before
3a   I have no appetite at all
3b   I crave food all of the time

19. Concentration Difficulties

0   I can concentrate as well as ever
1   I can't concentrate as well as usual
2   It's hard to keep my mind on anything for very long
3   I find I can't concentrate on anything

20. Tiredness or Fatigue

0   I am no more tired or fatigued than usual
1   I get more tired or fatigued more easily than usual
2   I am too tired or fatigued to do a lot of things I used to do
3   I am too tired or fatigued to do most of the things that I used to do

21. Loss of Interest in Sex

0   I have not noticed any recent change in my interest in sex
1   I am less interested in sex than I used to be
2   I am much less interested in sex now
3   I have lost in sex completely

BDI-II Scoring

Total Scores	Range
0 -13	Minimal
14 -19	Mild
20 – 28	Moderate
29- 63	Severe

DAST (Drug Abuse Screening Test)

1. Have you used drugs other than those required for medical reasons?	Yes	No
2. Have you abused prescription drugs?	Yes	No
3. Do you abuse more than one drug at a time?	Yes	No
4. Can you get through the week without using drugs (other than those required for medical reasons)?	Yes	No
5. Are you always able to stop using drugs when you want to?	Yes	No
6. Do you abuse drugs on a continuous basis?	Yes	No
7. Do you try to limit your drug use to certain situations?	Yes	No
8. Have you had "blackouts" or "flashbacks" as a result of drug use?	Yes	No
9. Do you ever feel bad about your drug abuse?	Yes	No
10. Does your spouse (or parents) ever complain about your involvement with drugs?	Yes	No
11. Do your friends or relatives know or suspect you abuse drugs?	Yes	No
12. Has drug abuse ever created problems between you and your spouse?	Yes	No
13. Has any family member ever sought help for problems related to your drug use?	Yes	No
14. Have you ever lost friends because of your use of drugs?	Yes	No
15. Have you ever neglected your family or missed work because of your use of drugs?	Yes	No
16. Have you ever been in trouble at work because of drug abuse?	Yes	No
17. Have you ever lost a job because of drug abuse?	Yes	No
18. Have you gotten into fights when under the influence of drugs?	Yes	No
19. Have you ever been arrested because of unusual behavior while under the influence of drugs?	Yes	No
20. Have you ever been arrested for driving while under the influence of drugs?	Yes	No
21. Have you engaged in illegal activities to obtain drugs?	Yes	No
22. Have you ever been arrested for possession of illegal drugs?	Yes	No
23. Have you ever experienced withdrawal symptoms as a result of heavy drug intake?	Yes	No
24. Have you had medical problems as a result of your drug use (e.g., memory loss, hepatitis, convulsions, or bleeding)?	Yes	No
25. Have you ever gone to anyone for help for a drug problem?	Yes	No
26. Have you ever been in hospital for medical problems related to your drug use?	Yes	No
27. Have you ever been involved in a treatment program specifically related to drug use?	Yes	No
28. Have you been treated as an outpatient for problems related to drug abuse?	Yes	No

Transition Planning

Proper Transition Planning has been identified as one of the factors that is most consistently correlated with positive outcomes in treatment. Treatment providers commonly observe that their clients do well while actively engaged in structured programming. Please note that the term "transition" replaces the more traditional "discharge" terminology. "Transition" seems to better capture the notion of continuity of care in a seamless system of services. We hope the Intervention Planner will encourage an examination and reformulation of traditional terminology for transitions in the continuum of care.

Respectfully, implementation of any set of guidelines is subject to the availability of resources and local circumstances. Community resources should be conceived of as an array of services and mutual supports which will operate as a unified system of care. If community resources are limited, the transition plan should make the most effective use of the resources that are available and reflect the most important priorities for the client in question. Realistic determinations should be made on a case by case basis. Ideally, transitions between levels of care will be based on clear criteria. Ultimately, ideal planning for level of care transitions can be achieved only through an integrated, client driven community based system of care.

Transition management is clearly a process rather than a discreet operation. The following principles for transition management are offered as elements of this process which will help to insure that service users are enabled to stay in treatment to the greatest extent possible.

Principles for Transition of Care Between Levels of Care

1. Prioritization: Transition planning should begin at the time of admission to any level of care and should be a prominent part of the treatment plan. Identification of transition needs and the coordination of services required to meet them will be most urgent and have greatest importance at the most intense levels of care.

2. Client Involvement: The client's wishes with regard to continuing care must be factored heavily into a transition plan. A plan that the client is not invested in is one that is not likely to succeed. While the service user's judgment may be questioned in the early stages of recovery, if the client cannot be persuaded and convinced of the wisdom of plans which do not coincide with their own thinking, efforts must be made to develop as constructive a plan as possible that takes into account the wishes and perceived needs of the client. Plans should focus on the service user's unique circumstances and should acknowledge and use their identified strengths.

3. Co-Morbidity: A significant percentage of individuals in addiction treatment settings have co-morbid psychiatric or medical conditions which require continuing care, but transition plans do not usually address these issues adequately. All addiction programs should develop policies for transition planning regarding psychiatric and medical illnesses that incorporate the principles listed here. Transition plans should routinely strive for *integrated* treatment of psychiatric and additive disorders and *collaborative* treatment of medical and addictive disorders for individuals with co-occurring disorders. Provisions should be made to ensure continuity even in the event of relapse, and to facilitate access to dual recovery peer supports.

4. Comprehensiveness: Transition plans should include all aspects of an individual's service needs. This type of comprehensive planning has not always been a part of traditional approaches to addiction treatment. Referral to treatment services alone have frequently been considered to be sufficient. Although substance use programs have traditionally not been funded as generously as mental health services, a multidimensional view of client needs must be considered and a full array of supportive services should be available to transition planners. These would typically include services such as case management, child care, residential stabilization, treatment of co-morbid issues of mental or physical health, realistic financial supports, and mutual support networking. In some cases interface with the legal system or child protection/family service agencies will be required.

5. Collaboration: Coordination of and collaboration between elements of the service system which are involved with the client on either side of the transition should occur as part of the treatment plan such that a sense of continuity is achieved while the transition evolves. It is helpful to think of a transition team when developing a transition plan, and this coordination must be elevated in status to an essential aspect of the transition plan, rather than an afterthought. Short of this, information regarding the most recent treatment experience should be provided to the agency where the client will be continuing care. Appropriate incentives for providers are an essential consideration in efforts to achieve these objectives.

6. Continuum of Responsibility: Systems should develop clear protocols delineating responsibility for care of clients in transition periods. In most cases responsibilities should incorporate redundancies between the referring and receiving agencies. These concurrent responsibilities will be more likely to ensure a smooth transition and prevent some of the discontinuations commonly observed in systems which do not contain overlaps between levels of care. Reimbursement arrangements should incentivize processes which incorporate concurrent responsibilities where appropriate, for the following transitions functions:
· Client demonstrates awareness of location, time, and contact person for next scheduled treatment session
· Client has access to prescribed medication and a sufficient quantity is available to allow uninterrupted use between physician contacts.
· Client is aware of the person(s) to contact should there be any difficulties with either obtaining or using medication during the transition period or with any other aspects of required services.
· Client is aware of contact person for arranging alterations in the original discharge plan should such changes become necessary.
· Client is aware of tracking plan and the process that will be initiated to re-engage him/her should unplanned alterations in the plan occur.

7. Continuity: Transitions, either upward or downward in the continuum of services, should incorporate relevant elements of any preexisting treatment plan. Treatment plans should be relevant to the entire course of an episode of illness/disability so that they can provide a degree of continuity in the context of change if properly elaborated and utilized.

8. Support System Involvement: The degree of family involvement will generally be dictated by the client's and the family's willingness to engage in the process. Efforts to obtain this participation should be a priority of the transition team as family members often play a critical role in the addiction drama. Other persons providing support in the community, such as a PCP or spiritual advisor, should be included as well if a client indicates a desire for their participation. Consensus on the plan will increase the likelihood that the various participants will maintain a commitment to the process.

9. Relapse Prevention Strategies: Discharge planning from residential settings to community settings should include comprehensive relapse prevention planning. Strategies to avoid re-initiating old, dysfunctional patterns of behavior should be identified as well as available community supports and treatment programming. Financial supports should be arranged in such a manner as to avoid undue pressure to misuse funds in destructive ways.

10. Pragmatism: Transition/Discharge plans must reflect reality and address client needs in the most practical way possible. This will require recognition of the phase of illness and/or recovery of the client for which services are being planned. In many cases, clients may choose to leave treatment early or they may have had marginal investment in the service they are departing from. Regardless of the circumstances of their departure or the likelihood of their continuing in treatment, a comprehensive plan should be elaborated in a manner which is as inclusive of client wishes as possible. The overall goal in many instances will be to minimize the potential for harmful outcomes. This objective may be particularly relevant to working with persons who have disabling mental disorders.

11. Maximize Resources: Transitions have frequently required that clients return to situations in which their basic needs are not adequately met. The transition/discharge plan should be designed to maximize the resources available to the client for continuing care. This includes efforts to secure benefits for which the client is eligible with the active participation of the client. Planning should foster self reliance while recognizing that significant support may be required in the early stages of recovery. Distinctions between enabling interventions and necessary supports should be consistently drawn and frequently scrutinized, but with a realization that an overly rigid, withholding approach is often counterproductive. This latter point is particularly relevant to work with persons who have co-occurring mental disorders.

12. Confidentiality: Information sharing should occur only in the context of client consent. Statutory requirements for confidential treatment of information related to addiction treatment are well understood by most clinicians, but clear consideration of these requirements with the client is important, and may assist in the establishment of trust in the transition planning process.

13. Cultural Sensitivity: Transitions should be managed in a culturally sensitive manner. Considering this in its broadest sense, an individual's beliefs, customs, and social context must be considered when making transitions upward (to more intensive levels of service) or downward (to less intensive levels of service).

14. Timing: Whenever possible, transitions should take place gradually, titrated according to an individual's ability to adapt to changing roles and expectations.

15. Quality Management: A mechanism for monitoring outcomes of transition plans and identifying opportunities to improve the process should be in place.
· Appropriate quality indicators should be established with realistic benchmarks which can be easily measured.
· A mechanism for establishing corrective action plans for systems unable to meet those expectations should be elaborated.

· Documentation should clearly indicate that all responsibilities delineated above occur and that they do so within appropriate time frames
· Oversight of the quality management process should include all stakeholders in the system, including persons in recovery.
· Standards established should be incorporated into contracts with Managed Care Organizations to assure proper incentives in reimbursement

Co-Occurring Psychiatric Disorders

There has been growing recognition that a very significant number of persons with substance use disorders suffer from concurrent psychiatric disorders. Substance use treatment programs must develop proficiency in assessing and treating these problems, just as mental health programs must be proficient in addressing substance use issues. Likewise, the transition plan must reflect the importance of addressing both illnesses adequately. The principles provided above will apply well to persons will Co-Occurring disorders, but when developing a service plan, additional issues may need to be considered:

These clients may require additional supports to engage with the treatment process beyond restrictive settings. Medication management is a significant concern when planning transitions, both in terms of continuity and with regard to acceptability of the plan.

Expectations of total abstinence may need to be tempered by harm reduction perspectives that provide some flexibility for addressing problems with ongoing substance use. Adopting this perspective may provide a basis for engagement and eventual investment in a change process.

Unique mutual support programs may be needed to address the issues relevant to the dual recovery client. Services must meet client needs rather than attempting to make clients fit into pre-existing programming.

Disclaimer

References

American Psychiatric Association. 1994. *Diagnostic and statistical manual of mental disorders, fourth edition*. Washington, DC: American Psychiatric Association, p. 176.

American Society of Addiction Medicine. 2001. *ASAM public policy statement: Treatment for alcoholism and other drug dependencies*. Posted at www.asam.org/ppol/treatment.htm.

Centers for Disease Control and Prevention. Additional recommendations to reduce sexual and drug-abuse related transmission of human Tlymphotropic virus type III/lymphadenopathy-associated virus. *Morb Mortal Wkly Rep* 35:152 - 155, 1986.

Chaney, E.F. Social skills training. In: Hester, R.K., and Miller, W.R., eds. *Handbook of Alcoholism Treatment Approaches: Effective Alternatives*. New York: Pergamon Press, 1989. pp. 206-221.

Crowley, T.J. Contingency contracting treatment of drug-abusing physicians, nurses, and dentists. In: Grabowski, J.; Stitzer, M.L.; and Henningfield, J.E., eds. *Behavioral Intervention Techniques in Drug Abuse Treatment. NIDA Research Monograph 46*. Pub. No. (ADM)84-1282. Rockville, MD: National Institute on Drug Abuse, 1984. pp. 68 - 83.

Daley KC. Update on Attention Deficit Hyperactivity Disorder. *Curr Opin Pediatr.* 2004 Apr;16(2):217-26.

Derogatis, L.R. *SCL-90R: Administration, Scoring and Procedures Manual - II*. Towson, MD: Clinical Psychometric Research, 1983.

deBeus R., Ball J.D., deBeus M.E., Herrington R. Attention training with ADHD children: preliminary findings in a double-blind placebo-controlled study. Presented at the Annual Conference of the International Society for Neuronal Regulation. Houston: August 29, 2003.

Gorski, Terence T., John M. Kelley, Lisa Havens, and Roger H. Peters. 1993. *Relapse prevention and the substance-abusing criminal offender: Technical assistance publication series 8*. Rockville, MD: Department of Health and Human Services, Substance Abuse and Mental Health Services Administration, p. 9.

Selzer, M.L. The Michigan Alcoholism Screening Test: The quest for a new diagnostic instrument. *Am J Psychiatry* 127(12):1653 - 1658, 1971.

Shaner, A.; Roberts, L.J.; Eckman, T.A.; Tucker, D.E.; Tsuang, J.W.; Wilkins, J.N.; and Mintz, J. Monetary reinforcement of abstinence from cocaine among mentally ill patients with cocaine dependence. *Psychiatr Serv* 48(6):807 - 810, 1997.

Silverman, K.; Higgins, S.T.; Brooner, R.K.; Montoya, I.D.; Cone, E.J.; Schuster, C.R.; and Preston, K.L. Sustained cocaine abstinence in methadone maintenance patients through voucher-based reinforcement theory. *Arch Gen Psychiatry* 53(5):409 - 415, 1996.

Silverman, K.; Wong, C.J.; Higgins, S.T.; Brooner, R.K.; Montoya, I.D.; Contoreggi, C.; Umbricht-Schneiter, A.; Schuster, C.R.; and Preston, K.L. Increasing opiate abstinence through voucher-based reinforcement therapy. Drug Alcohol Depend 41(2):157 - 165, 1996.

Sisson, R., and Azrin, N.H. The community reinforcement approach. In: Hester, R.K., and Miller, W.R., eds. Handbook of Alcoholism Treatment Approaches: Effective Alternatives. New York: Pergamon Press, 1989. pp. 242 - 258.

Sobell, L.C.; Sobell, M.B.; Leo, G.I.; and Cancilla, A. Reliability of a timeline method: Assessing normal drinkers' reports of recent drinking and a comparative evaluation across several populations. Br J Addict 83(4):393 - 402, 1988.

Sulzer-Azaroff, B., and Meyer, G.R. Behavior Analysis for Lasting Change. Fort Worth, TX: Holt Rinehart and Winston, 1991.

Tusel, D.J.; Piotrowski, N.A.; Sees, K.; Reilly, P.M.; Banys, P.; Meek, P.; and Hall, S.M. Contingency contracting for illicit drug use with opioid addicts in methadone treatment. In: Harris, L.S., ed. Problems of Drug Dependence, 1994: Proceedings of the 56th Annual Scientific Meeting. National Institute on Drug Abuse Research Monograph 153. Washington, DC: Supt. of Docs., U.S. Govt. Print. Off., 1995. pp. 155 - 160.

Special Reference Resource

Diagnostic and Statistical Manual of Mental Disorders-Forth Addition-Text Revision (DSM-IV-TR)

Additional Books Written
by this Author
Listed and Sold Exclusively on Amazon

- Treatment Planning Guide for Substance Abuse/Mental Health Services

- A Clinicians' Guide to Writing Successful Treatment Plans

- A Clinicians' Guide to Writing Successful Treatment Plans
  (Desk Top Version)

- Early Drug Education   Grades 1 - 6

- Drug Education and Awareness Program   Workbooks 1 - 6

- Drug Education and Awareness   Exp. Workbooks 1 - 6
  (Includes Rational and Learning objectives)

- Pre-Teen Drug Education and Awareness Program   Man./Workbooks 1 - 6
  (For Facilitator/Therapist use)

- Teen Drug Education and Awareness Program   Complete Program

- Addiction and Recovery Management   (Book 1)
  Successful Tools for a Creative Recovery

- Addiction and Recovery   (Book 2)
  Addiction Advice that Could Save Your Life

- Prevent Bullying   Complete Program
  (Facilitators Guide for School Age Children)

About the Author

Ramsey Bradley, M.S., holds a Master's Degree in Counseling and Psychology, a Bachelor's Degree in Education having graduated with Phi Theta Kappa Honors. He has more than 28 years of experience working in private practice and public mental health/substance abuse settings.

Throughout his career as a therapist, a business owner, and Director of Outpatient Clinical Programs, Ramsey has developed many therapeutic programs that have been certified by the Florida Department of Children and Families as "Researched Based" programs under their "Best Practices".

Currently Ramsey resides in Cocoa Beach, Florida. He now finds time out of his busy schedule writing books pertaining to Substance Abuse and Mental Health issues in his continued effort to hopefully reach people who may need help and support during life's ups and downs.

You will find that all of his books are sold exclusively on Amazon.com- Just search on Amazon for-Ramsey Bradley MS.

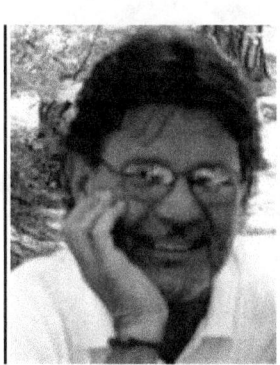

www.ingramcontent.com/pod-product-compliance
Lightning Source LLC
Chambersburg PA
CBHW081602220526
45468CB00010B/2744